CORE
Stability

On The Ball

researched and written by

Karen Petko B.A., KIN (Hons)

photography by

Suzanne Maunder

published by

Trafford Publishing Ltd.

disclaimer

No manual or book can adequately replace the services of a trained physician, certified kinesiologist or other qualified health or exercise professional. Any application of the information set out or described in this manual is done at the reader's discretion and risk.

Order this book online at www.trafford.com
or email orders@trafford.com

Most Trafford titles are also available at major online book retailers.

Print information available on the last page.

ISBN: 978-1-4120-5934-3 (sc)
ISBN: 978-1-4122-3646-1 (e)

Trafford rev. 02/08/2019

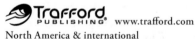 www.trafford.com

North America & international
toll-free: 1 888 232 4444 (USA & Canada)
fax: 812 355 4082

table of contents

introduction

The Stability or Swiss Ball is an effective tool that offers unlimited training possibilities for healthy as well as disabled individuals. By training on a Stability Ball you are able to strengthen your back, improve your posture and define overall muscle tone.

The Exercise Ball is a challenging training device that provides a new dimension: *instability*. This unique characteristic strengthens and stretches every muscle of the body in an effective way. When exercising with an Exercise Ball you need to maintain proper body alignment and good technique by contracting deep core stabilizing muscles. Muscles you have never worked before are now being challenged in order to maintain proper posture and balance on the ball.

Simply, the Stability Ball is a challenging and functional training device. When used correctly, the Stability Ball can strengthen your body as a whole unit by improving muscular balance and enhancing functional movements.

This manual contains both *strengthening exercises* and *flexibility stretches* for your core musculature (abdominals, low back and gluteal/hip muscles). Research has shown that strengthening these deep core muscles will help avoid excessively loading or irritating our spinal discs, joints and ligaments. Poor core strength can lead to muscle imbalances, a higher risk for injuries as well as back pain.

With this manual, you will learn the proper starting positions, alignment, execution and progressions of specific therapeutic exercises for your core muscles. It is extremely important to follow the instructions and pictures of each exercise as closely as possible. For exercises with progressions, start with the Basic Level until you develop more strength to progress to the Advanced Level. Enjoy and get on the ball!

safety tips

1. It is a good idea to consult your physician before beginning any type of exercise program. Some of the exercises could affect a medical condition especially if you have high blood pressure, glaucoma, a joint condition, osteoporosis or are pregnant. If you experience any pain, cramping, dizziness, nausea or discomfort while exercising with the stability ball stop the exercises immediately and consult your physician.

2. Read the instructions carefully before each exercise and follow the pictures as closely as possible for the proper body positions.

3. For exercises that have progressions, start with the Basic Level until you have mastered the exercise and have developed enough strength to progress to the Advanced Level.

4. Inspect your stability ball prior to each workout to ensure that there are no scratches or cuts. If your ball is damaged discontinue use immediately.

5. Avoid exercising with your stability ball on slippery surfaces.

general guidelines

precautions

• If you experience any pain, cramping, dizziness, nausea or discomfort while exercising stop the exercises immediately and consult your physician.

• Do not eat prior to your workout. Allow at least 2 hours after eating depending upon the size of the meal before exercising.

• Exercise in an area free of obstructions.

• Comfortable tight fitted clothing is recommended.

• Remember to breathe properly.

sizing tips

• Ball sizes are categorized according to one's height.

• In general, when seated on the ball your knees should be level with or slightly above your hips; thighs should be parallel with the floor and knees should be bent at a 90-degree angle.

inflation tips & ball care

• Your ball can be inflated using a normal bike pump or gas station pump.

• Inflate your ball to the point when it becomes firm but has some give to it; this will allow the ball to conform to your body shape.

• To clean use mild soapy water.

• Keep your stability ball away from sunlight and intense heat.

benefits of stability ball training

Swiss or Stability Balls are large, colorful, inflated beach balls that were originally used in the 1960's by Swiss physical therapists for orthopedic rehabilitation. Their popularity has grown tremendously over the past few years. These Stability Balls are now being used in physiotherapy clinics for rehabilitation as well as in the fitness industry to improve and prevent back disorders.

Your core muscles - abdominals, hip/gluteal and back-stabilize your entire body. It is important to strengthen deep abdominal and back muscles that brace and support the spine. This solid foundation increases your ability to function with everyday activities. The balance between the muscles of the abdomen and back can be achieved effectively while training with a Stability Ball.

The benefits/advantages of the Stability Ball are endless:

- instability of the ball challenges overall balance
- entire body must work to stabilize
- allows you to train in a multi-planar environment
- helps build functional strength
- spherical shape provides an increased range of motion for flexibility
- focuses on hard-to-get-to muscles=deep postural muscles (transverse abdominis, erector spinae)
- strengthening these core muscles prevents further injury and relieves back pain
- improves overall balance, coordination, posture, strength and flexibility

In essence, strength training on the ball results in a strong and stable core. Having a strong core enables you to stabilize your spine as you move, lift and respond in an ever-changing environment.

benefits

stability ball principles

The stability ball is an innovative fitness tool that provides sensational results. It incorporates strength training with postural awareness and overall coordination training. The basic principles involved when using this fitness tool are:

- instability
- lever length
- positioning

instability

Training with an exercise ball offers a new dimension: instability. This challenging feature provides you with an unstable base of support and targets deep abdominal muscle training, postural awareness and overall balance.

lever length

The intensity of an exercise may be increased or decreased by altering the lever length= the distance between your body and the stability ball. For example, the closer the stability ball is to your midsection the easier the exercise will be; the farther away the stability ball is from your midsection the more difficult the exercise will be.

positioning

When training with a stability ball the positioning varies from exercise to exercise (supine, prone, seated, upright, feet elevated). This is a great advantage over using a traditional workout bench because of the increased challenge and deep abdominal muscle recruitment.

principles

anatomy 101

core muscles

• Set of deep postural muscles responsible for maintaining proper posture and body alignment

abdominal wall muscle group

• **rectus abdominis:** "six-pack" muscle responsible for lumbar flexion
• **external obliques:** largest most superficial muscle responsible for lumbar flexion and rotation
• **internal obliques:** lies between external obliques and transverse abdominis
• **transverse abdominis:** deepest abdominal muscle responsible for spinal stability

back muscle group

• **erector spinae:** group of deep muscles that run along the vertebral column responsible for lumbar extension
• **multifidus:** series of deep muscles that contribute to low back and pelvic stability
• **lattisimus dorsi:** large superficial muscle responsible for low back extension
• **thoracolumbar fascia:** three layers of connective tissue critical in stabilizing the trunk
• **quadratus lumborum:** deep muscle responsible for stabilizing the lumbar spine

gluteal muscle group

• **gluteus maximus**: very powerful muscle that provides control and stability for the low back

Performing strengthening exercises that target all of these muscle groups will help build a strong and stable torso. Emphasis should be placed on practicing torso stabilization. Training these core muscles will help form a tight inner unit enabling proper body posture and alignment. If this unit is not functioning properly, other muscles will be exhausted placing excessive wear and tear on our joints and ligaments. Core stability is the answer to a healthy pain free back.

anatomy

orientation & lumbar mobility

neutral position

focus
Used as a starting position for many exercises.

- Sit on the ball as if you are on a chair.
- Feet should be shoulder width apart with knees bent at 90 degrees.
- Ribcage and chest are high with shoulders down and back.

trainer's tip:
Lengthen your spine and practice setting your abdominals.

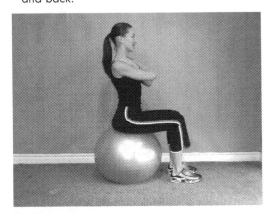

pelvic tilts

focus
To increase lumbar mobility by reducing muscular and joint stiffness in the low back. Also increases abdominal tone.

starting position
Assume neutral position.

- Allow the ball to roll forward tightening your abdominal muscles and flattening your back.
- Movement should occur only at the pelvis.

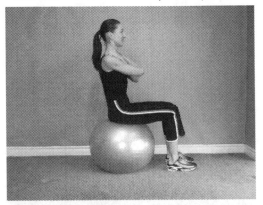

lumbar mobility

lateral tilts

focus
To increase lumbar mobility by reducing muscular and joint stiffness in the low back.

starting position
Assume neutral position.

- Tilt hips to one side allowing the ball to roll.
- Return back to neutral position.
- Keep your body tall and allow movement to occur only at the pelvis.

trainer's tip:
Perform a slow and controlled tilt allowing your back muscles to release and relax.

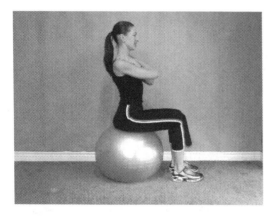

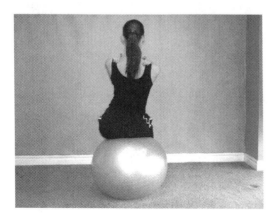

lumbar mobility

basic walkout

focus
To increase coordination, body awareness and overall balance.

starting position
Assume neutral position.

- Walk your feet out allowing your back to roll down the ball.
- Return to a seated position by walking your feet back and curling your trunk forward.

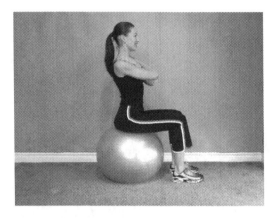

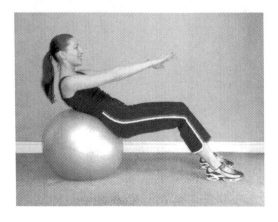

seated on the ball

balance work

focus
To improve core control and overall balance.

starting position
Assume neutral position.

- Set your abdominals.
- Lift one foot off the floor.
- Repeat with other leg.

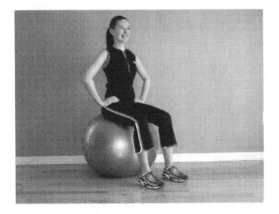

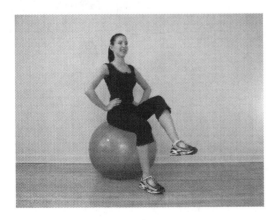

seated on the ball

torso stabilization

setting your abdominals

Your anatomical girdle consists of your core muscles:

- abdominals (rectus abdominis, transverse abdominis, internal/external obliques)
- low back (erector spinae, multifidus, latissimus dorsi, thoracolumbar fascia, quadratus lumborum)
- gluteal/hip (gluteus maximus/medius)

This girdle provides protection for your spine during any type of activity. It helps to maintain or stabilize your body's equilibrium as it moves.

Unfortunately, the core is often ignored or not targeted properly. Repeated core muscle training reinforces muscle memory patterns as well as proper muscle recruitment. As day to day living involves constant change, your body is continuously being challenged to react to its dynamic environment.

To improve the strength and function of your anatomical girdle, a simple yet important technique is used prior to each strengthening exercise executed with a Stability Ball. This technique is known as *'setting your abdominals'* and can be achieved by drawing your navel (bellybutton) in towards your spine. This setting action should be gentle and controlled. By practicing this exercise your deep core muscles contract and help stabilize your spine. This initiation of your inner unit acts as a support system for your back and torso.

focus
To initiate an inner unit contraction.

starting position
Assume neutral position. Inhale to prepare, as you exhale pull your bellybutton in towards your spine. Hold for 5 seconds. Repeat 8-12 times.

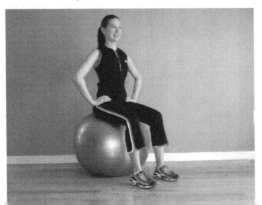

cardiovascular exercise

- It is important to warm-up and raise your core temperature prior to every workout. This increases the blood flow to the muscles and loosens the tissues ready to work. Your muscles and joints will be warm and ready to go.
- You may accomplish this with your favorite video warm-up or if your have access to any cardio equipment such as a treadmill, stationary bike or elliptical trainer.
- Remember to exercise at a comfortable pace. You should be able to maintain a conversation while exercising.
- Cardiovascular exercise (20-40 minutes) performed at least 3 times a week will increase your energy level, burn calories and improve overall fitness.

core strengthening exercises

- Each position should be held for 5 seconds.
- Each exercise should be performed in sets of 2-3 with 8-12 repetitions of each. For example, perform 10 reps of one exercise, take a brief break and then perform another 10 reps of the same exercise. Repeat this with each strengthening exercise.
- Remember to 'Set Your Abdominals' before each exercise.

breathing technique

Slow and controlled breathing is extremely important when exercising.

With every exercise:

- inhale to prepare
- exhale as you execute the exercise
- inhale and hold the desired position
- exhale and release

cardio tips

supine tabletop

focus
To increase body awareness and improve core control.

starting position
Assume neutral position.

- Walk your feet out allowing your back to roll down on the ball.
- Keep your head and shoulders supported on the ball.
- Hips are held high level with your body.
- Return back up to neutral position by walking your feet back and curling your trunk up.
- Hold the tabletop position for 5 seconds. Repeat 8-12 times.

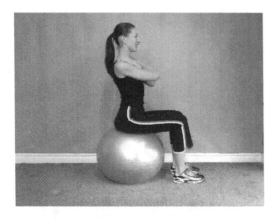

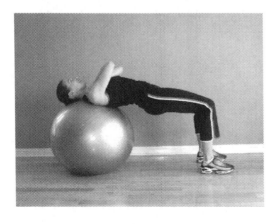

supine on the ball

tabletop hip drops

focus
To strengthen abdominal and gluteal muscle groups and improve overall balance.

starting position
Assume tabletop position with arms crossed over chest.

- Drop your hips to the floor keeping your head and shoulders supported on the ball.
- Lift your hips back up level with your body to the tabletop position.
- Hold position for 5 seconds. Repeat 8-12 times.

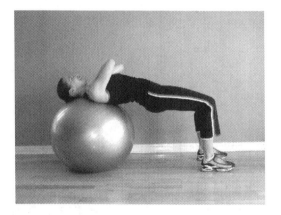

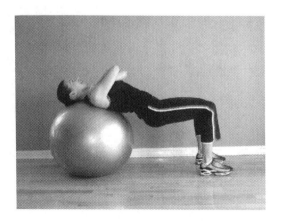

supine on the ball

advanced hip drops

starting position
From the tabletop position, cross one leg over the other.

- Drop your hips to the floor keeping your head and shoulders supported on the ball.
- Lift your hips back up level with your body to the tabletop position.
- Hold position for 5 seconds. Repeat 8-12 times.

trainer's tip:
Keep your chest high with knees stacked over your ankles.

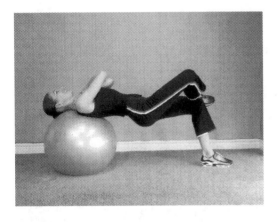

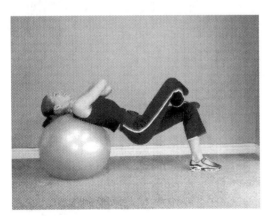

supine on the ball

torso curls

focus
To increase abdominal strength and improve overall balance.

starting position
From neutral position, walk your feet out until your back is supported on the ball. Cross your arms over your chest.

- Pull your ribs towards your hips curling your trunk.
- Lift both shoulders off the ball.
- Avoid pulling on the head or neck.
- Repeat 8-12 times.

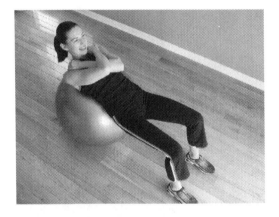

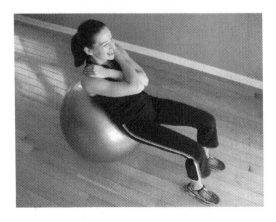

abs on the ball

advanced torso curls

starting position

From neutral position, walk your feet out until your body is further back on the ball (this increases the difficulty of the exercise). Place both hands behind your head.

- Pull your ribs towards your hips curling your trunk.
- Lift both shoulders off the ball.
- Avoid pulling on the head or neck.
- Repeat 8-12 times.

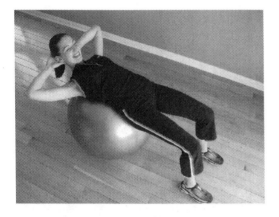

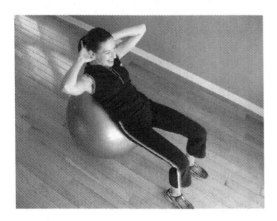

abs on the ball

torso twists

focus
To increase abdominal strength (specifically the oblique muscles) and improve overall balance.

starting position
From neutral position, walk your feet out until your back is supported on the ball. Cross your arms over your chest.

- Pull your ribs towards your hips curling your trunk and twisting to one side (left shoulder to right hip).
- Avoid pulling on your head or neck.
- Alternate twists to both sides.
- Repeat 8-12 times.

trainer's tip:
Remember to set your abdominals prior to and during each twist. Do not hold your breath.

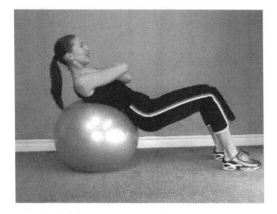

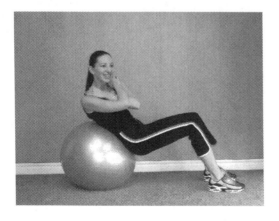

abs on the ball

advanced torso twists

starting position

From neutral position, walk your feet out until your body is further back on the ball.

- Pull your ribs towards your hips curling your trunk and twisting to one side (left shoulder to right hip).
- Avoid pulling on your head or neck.
- Alternate twists to both sides.
- Repeat 8-12 times.

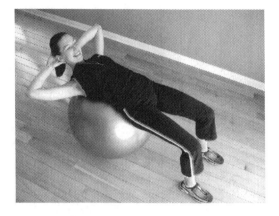

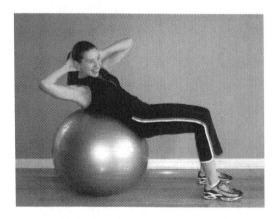

abs on the ball

modified torso curls

focus
To increase abdominal strength.

starting position
Lying supine, place the ball under your calves.

- Pull your ribs towards your hips curling your trunk.
- Lift both shoulders off the floor.
- Flex both knees.
- Avoid pulling on your head or neck.
- Repeat 8-12 times.

trainer's tip:
Remember to set your abdominals prior to and during each curl. Breathe properly.

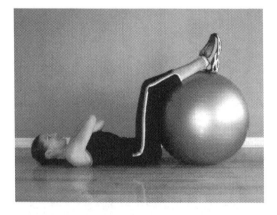

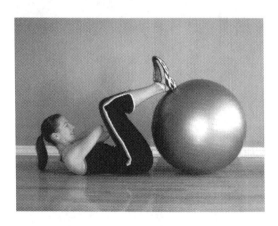

feet elevated on the ball

modified torso twists

focus
To increase abdominal strength (specifically the oblique muscles).

starting position
Lying supine, place the ball under your calves.

- Pull your ribs towards your hips curling your trunk and twisting to one side.
- Avoid pulling on the head or neck.
- Flex both knees.
- Alternate twists to both sides.
- Repeat 8-12 times.

trainer's tip:
Do not hold your breath: inhale to prepare, exhale as you crunch up, inhale on the release.

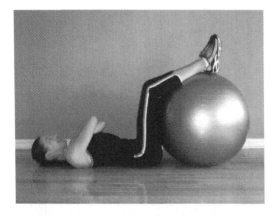

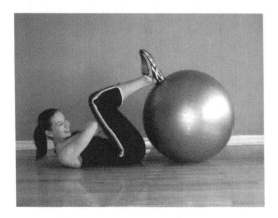

feet elevated on the ball

basic bridging

focus
To strengthen the abdominal, low back and gluteal muscle groups. Also improves overall balance.

starting position
Lying supine with ball under your calves and hands by your sides.

- Set your abdominals.
- Lift your hips up towards the ceiling.
- Hold this position for 5 seconds. Repeat 8-12 times.
- Keep the ball stable throughout the exercise.

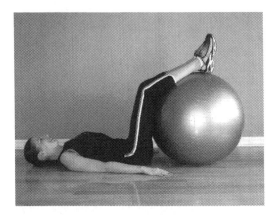

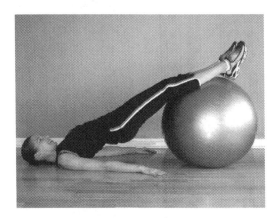

feet elevated on the ball

advanced bridging

starting position

Lying supine, place the ball under your ankles with arms crossed over your chest.

- Set your abdominals.
- Lift your hips up towards the ceiling.
- Hold this position for 5 seconds. Repeat 8-12 times.
- Keep the ball stable throughout the exercise.

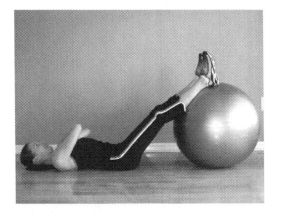

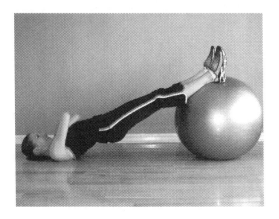

feet elevated on the ball

ultimate bridging

focus
To strengthen abdominal, low back, gluteal and inner thigh muscle groups.

starting position
Lying supine, place the ball in between your shins with knees slightly flexed.

- Set your abdominals.
- As your lift your hips up towards the ceiling, squeeze the ball between your legs.
- Hold this position for 5 seconds. Repeat 8-12 times.

trainer's tip:
This is a challenging exercise that should be attempted <u>only</u> when Basic Bridging & Advanced Bridging have been fully mastered.

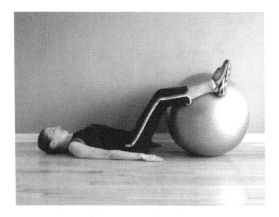

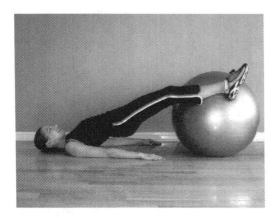

feet elevated on the ball

supine hamstring curls

focus
To strengthen the hamstring muscle group.

starting position
Lying supine, place the ball under your ankles with legs partially extended.

- Push the heels of both feet into the ball and roll the ball in towards your torso.
- Hold this position for 5 seconds.
- Extend the legs outward keeping the heels pressed into the ball.
- Repeat 8-12 times.

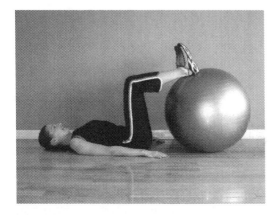

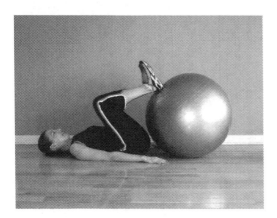

feet elevated on the ball

supermans

focus

To strengthen the mid and low back muscle groups. Also improves overall balance and coordination.

starting position

Lying prone over the ball, hands should be under the shoulders with knees under the hips and back straight.

- With knees in contact with the floor, extend one arm with the opposite leg until your limbs are parallel with the floor.
- Hold this position for 5 seconds.
- Release and switch sides.
- Repeat 8-12 times.

trainer's tip:
Think of lengthening your arm and leg rather than lifting up. Keep your head in neutral to avoid straining your neck.

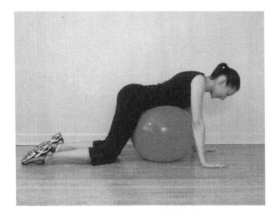

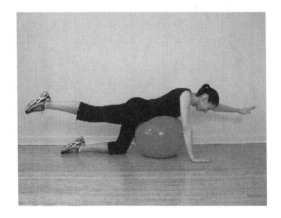

prone on the ball

advanced supermans

starting position

Lying prone over the ball, extend the legs so both knees are off the floor.

- With knees off the floor, extend one arm with the opposite leg until your limbs are parallel with the floor.
- Hold this position for 5 seconds.
- Release and switch sides.
- Repeat 8-12 times.

trainer's tip:
Remember to set your abdominals to support and stabilize your spine prior to each repetition.

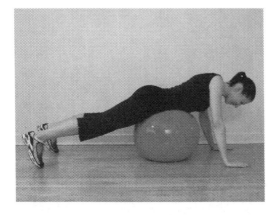

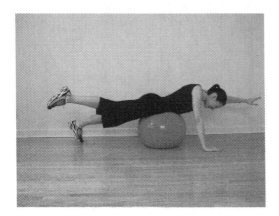

prone on the ball

prone trunk extensions

focus
To strengthen the low back muscle groups (spinal extensors).

starting position
Lying prone over the ball with knees flexed on the mat.

- With arms on the small of your back, straighten your spine lifting your chest off the ball.
- Hold position for 5 seconds. Repeat 8-12 times.

trainer's tip:
Pelvis should stay stable with your head and neck held in neutral position.

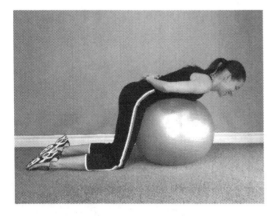

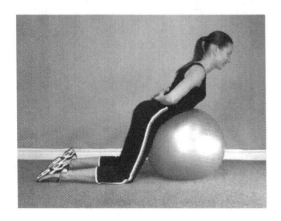

prone on the ball

prone trunk rotations

focus
To strengthen the low back muscle groups (spinal rotators).

starting position
Lying prone over the ball with knees flexed on the mat.

- With one arm on the ball and the other at your temple, straighten your spine and rotate to one side.
- Hold position for 5 seconds. Repeat 8-12 times.
- Keep pelvis stable with head and neck in neutral.

trainer's tip:
Movement should be diagonal and performed in a fluid and controlled manner.

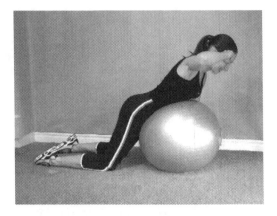

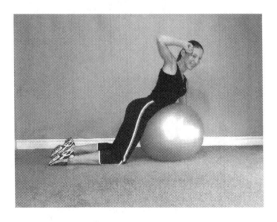

prone on the ball

prone walkout

focus
To strengthen the core muscle groups and improve overall balance.

starting position
Lying prone over the ball.

- Use both hands to walk out allowing the ball to roll along the body.
- Hold the position with the ball under your knees for 5 seconds.
- Slowly walk the hands back to starting position.
- Repeat 8-12 times.

trainer's tip:
Remember to set your abdominals to support and stabilize your spine throughout the entire exercise.

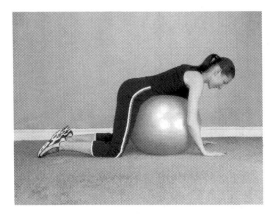

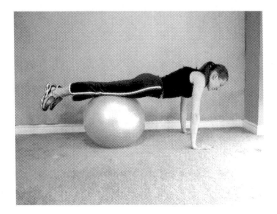

prone on the ball

advanced prone walkout

starting position
Lying prone over the ball.

- Use both hands to walk out allowing the ball to roll past your knees until it reaches your ankles.
- Hold this position 5 seconds.
- Slowly walk the hands back to starting position.
- Repeat 8-12 times.

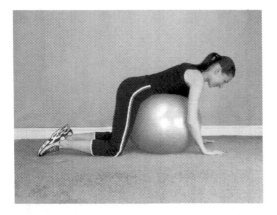

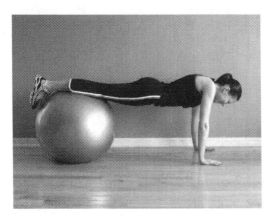

prone on the ball

prone push ups

focus
To improve core muscle and upper body strength.

starting position
Lying prone over the ball.

- Use both hands to walk out allowing the ball to position under your knees.
- Set your abdominals to support your spine.
- Perform a push up: bend both arms lowering your chest to the floor.
- Repeat 8-12 times.
- Slowly walk the hands back to starting position.

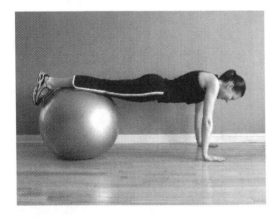

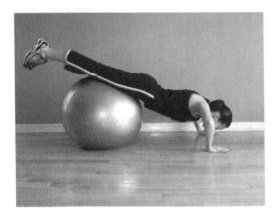

prone on the ball

wall squats

focus
To strengthen the gluteal, quadriceps and hamstring muscle groups.

starting position
Position the ball in the small of your back against the wall. Feet should be shoulder width apart and slightly away from the wall.

- Set your abdominals.
- Keeping your chest high, squat down until your thighs are almost parallel with the floor.
- As you squat push your gluteals back as if to sit on a chair.
- Hold position for 5 seconds. Repeat 8-12 times.

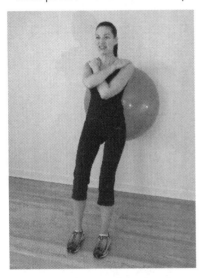

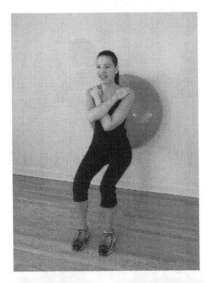

upright with the ball

wall lunges

focus
To strengthen the gluteal, quadriceps and hamstring muscle groups.

starting position
Assume same starting position as in previous exercise but anchor one foot back against the wall.

- Set your abdominals.
- Lower your body allowing the ball to roll against the wall.
- Lunge down until front knee is almost parallel to the floor.
- Hold position for 5 seconds. Repeat 8-12 times.

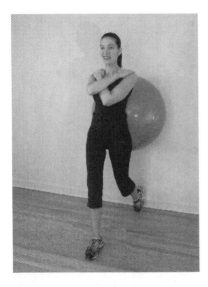

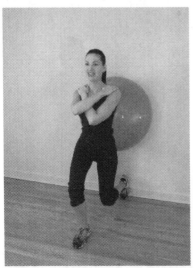

upright with the ball

flexibility stretches

Flexibility stretching involves the lengthening of muscles, tendons and ligaments. These soft tissues may become tight or tense due to injury, poor posture or repetitive motions. Stretching is essential for any workout because by increasing overall flexibility, it allows your muscles to move freely without any pain, tightness or discomfort.

Flexibility has endless benefits:
• reduces the risk of injury
• reduces muscle tension/soreness
• enhances overall body awareness
• increases mental and physical relaxation
• improves overall circulation

stretching formula

• Each stretch should be held for 30 seconds and repeated 3-5 times.
• Each stretch should be performed in a controlled and fluid manner with no bouncing or jerky movements.
• Muscles should be stretched to a comfortable point of pull with no pain.
• Remember to stretch with slow and controlled breathing.

breathing technique

Slow and controlled breathing is extremely important when stretching.
With every stretch:
• inhale to prepare
• exhale as you adopt the desired position
• inhale and hold the desired position
• exhale and release

stretching guidelines

lumbar flexion

focus
To stretch the low back muscle group and relieve tension on the lumbar spine.

starting position
Lying supine, place both feet on the ball.

- Roll the ball towards your trunk flexing your knees into your chest.
- Hold a comfortable stretch for 30 seconds.
- Repeat 3-5 times.

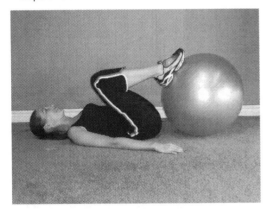

lumbar rotations

focus
To stretch the mid/low back and gluteal muscle groups by adopting a comfortable body twist.

starting position
Lying supine, reposition the ball under your knees.

- Keeping your head and shoulders on the mat, let your knees fall to one side.
- Hold a comfortable stretch for 30 seconds.
- Repeat to other side.

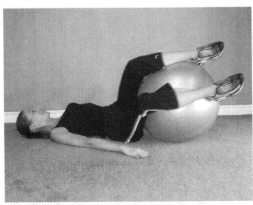

flexibility stretches

supine hamstring stretch

focus
To stretch the hamstring/calf muscle groups.

starting position
Lying supine with legs over the ball.

- Place your hands behind one leg.
- Straighten the leg up to the ceiling keeping the foot flexed.
- Hold a comfortable stretch for 30 seconds.
- Repeat with other leg.

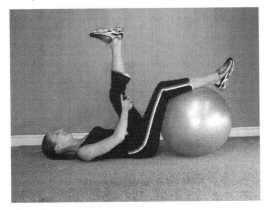

supine glute stretch

focus
To stretch the gluteal/hip muscle groups.

starting position
Lying supine with both feet on the ball.

- Cross one leg over the other, rolling the ball towards your trunk.
- Keep your knee flexed and hips on the mat.
- Hold a comfortable stretch for 30 seconds.
- Repeat with other leg.

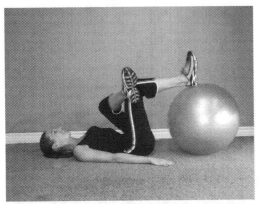

trainer's tip:
Tension in the hamstring and gluteal muscle groups lead to low back problems. Make sure you perform each stretch in a slow and controlled manner.

flexibility stretches

body arch stretch

focus
To stretch and relax the spinal muscles. Also assists with spine alignment reducing compression on the discs, joints and ligaments.

starting position
Begin in seated neutral position.

- Walk your feet out allowing the ball to roll under your spine.
- Rest your head on the ball as you let your arms fall to the floor.
- Hold a comfortable stretch for 30 seconds.
- Repeat 3-5 times.

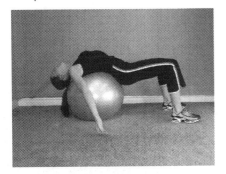

prone traction

focus
To release back tension, stimulate blood flow and enhance relaxation.

starting position
Lying prone over the ball.

- Center your trunk over the ball with hands crossed and feet on the floor.
- Relax and breathe in a slow and controlled manner.
- Hold a comfortable stretch for 30 seconds.
- Repeat 3-5 times.

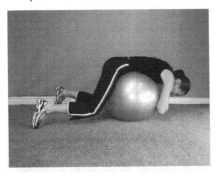

flexibility stretches

kneeling trunk stretch

focus
To stretch the upper/mid and lower back muscle groups.

starting position
Kneeling on the mat with hands on the ball.

- Roll the ball forward while sitting on your heels.
- Lengthen your torso.
- Hold a comfortable stretch for 30 seconds.
- Repeat 3-5 times.

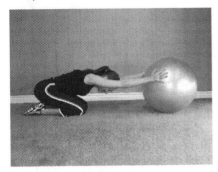

hip flexor stretch

focus
To stretch the hip flexor muscle group.

starting position
Begin kneeling on one knee.

- Holding the ball high, gently lean forward.
- Keep your trunk straight and ensure your front knee does not pass your toes.
- Hold a comfortable stretch for 30 seconds.
- Repeat with other leg.

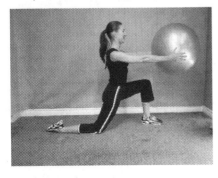

flexibility stretches

seated torso stretch

focus
To stretch the mid/low back muscle groups.

starting position
Begin in seated neutral position.

- Shift your weight to one side using your hand to counterbalance.
- Stretch the one hand up and over reaching for the ceiling.
- Hold a comfortable stretch for 30 seconds.
- Repeat to other side.

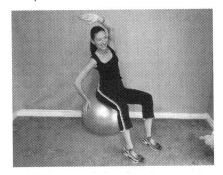

seated back stretch

focus
To stretch the mid/low back and hip muscle groups.

starting position
Begin in a seated neutral position.

- With legs comfortably bent, flex the spine forward.
- Let your upper body, hands and head rest comfortably.
- Hold a comfortable stretch for 30 seconds.
- Repeat 3-5 times.

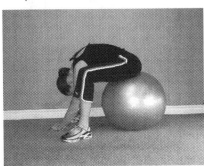

flexibility stretches

inner thigh stretch

focus
To stretch the inner thigh/hip muscle groups.

starting position
Adopt a comfortable stance with feet wider than shoulder width apart and hands resting on the ball.

- Shift your weight to one side; allowing the opposite leg to extend.
- Let the ball support your body weight.
- Hold a comfortable stretch for 30 seconds.
- Repeat to other side.

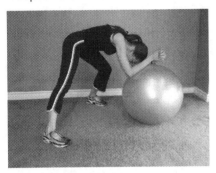

pike stretch

focus
To stretch the mid/low back, hamstring and gluteal muscle groups.

starting position
Feet should be shoulder width apart with hands on the ball.

- Roll the ball forward supporting your body weight on the ball.
- Keep the legs straight.
- Hold a comfortable stretch for 30 seconds.
- Repeat 3-5 times.

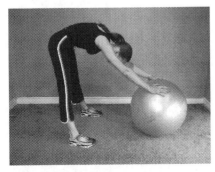

flexibility stretches

workout log

- plan your routine 3x a week every other day.
- choose exercises that challenge all of the muscles of your torso (abdominals, gluteal/hip and low back muscle groups).
- quality is more important than quantity.

short term goals

- prevent further injury
- improve muscular strength/overall flexibility

long term goals

- lose weight/burn calories
- improve overall health/well-being

cardiovascular warm-up

- treadmill walking
- stationary bike
- elliptical
- other

workout log

		S	M	T	W	T	F	S
CARDIO								
MOBILITY EXERCISES								
STRENGTH EXERCISES	# OF REPS							
FLEXIBILITY EXERCISES	# OF REPS							

		S	M	T	W	T	F	S
CARDIO								
MOBILITY EXERCISES								
STRENGTH EXERCISES	# OF REPS							
FLEXIBILITY EXERCISES	# OF REPS							

		S	M	T	W	T	F	S
CARDIO								
MOBILITY EXERCISES								
STRENGTH EXERCISES	# OF REPS							
FLEXIBILITY EXERCISES	# OF REPS							

		S	M	T	W	T	F	S
CARDIO								
MOBILITY EXERCISES								
STRENGTH EXERCISES	# OF REPS							
FLEXIBILITY EXERCISES	# OF REPS							

Printed in the United States
By Bookmasters